Autism Options Galore! 2006

Directory For Parents, Teachers And Professionals

By

Rosalie Seymour

Bloomington, IN  Milton Keynes, UK

authorHOUSE

AuthorHouse™
1663 Liberty Drive, Suite 200
Bloomington, IN 47403
www.authorhouse.com
Phone: 1-800-839-8640

AuthorHouse™ UK Ltd.
500 Avebury Boulevard
Central Milton Keynes, MK9 2BE
www.authorhouse.co.uk
Phone: 08001974150

First published by AuthorHouse 6/13/2006

ISBN: 1-4208-9553-2 (sc)

Printed in the United States of America
Bloomington, Indiana

This book is printed on acid-free paper.

ACKNOWLEGEMENTS

There was a time when I took my information from the people around me, professionals to whom I looked for direction and update. Then in 1993 I had the great fortune to attend a conference of the Geneva Centre in Toronto, and had the 'lid blown off' ' my mind through exposure to the wealth of information available. It was an intensely painful experience to realise that I had effectively been kept in the dark and thereby in blissful, 'don't rock the boat' mediocrity.

Since this time I have dedicated my efforts to empowering with information as many people in the field, parents and professionals, as possible. This course of action has generally been as well-received as Thomas Alva Edison at a candle makers' convention (to quote Annabel Stehli). Often I have been accused of giving parents 'false hope', as though there were such a thing!

There are those who fear new information. Nevertheless, increasing numbers of parents first, then professionals, are embracing the new developments that offer hope of improved outcomes for these children.

It is to you that I dedicate this work.

I wish to thank all those whose encouragement and suggestions kept me working on this directory, particularly Carin Smit , Hazel Trudgill and Dr Rosa Lewis. I would also like to acknowledge my colleagues, the speech and language therapists of Ireland, whose dedication and expertise are a constant inspiration. Thanks also to Kirsten Seymour who lent her expertise to the layout of this book.

In gratitude to the Lord of little children and lost lambs.

DISCLAIMER

The various intervention options presented in this directory are meant to be <u>only for the purpose of information.</u>

The topics are included for the sole purpose of informing readers that they exist.

This directory is in no way intended to serve as a recommendation of the suitability of any intervention in all nor any particular case.

The author cannot therefore be held responsible for the consequences of any action taken by any individual or group upon reading this material.

FOREWORD

This booklet is intended to serve as a handy carry-about diary and notebook. This might be the volume the reader can have in their bag as they visit the doctor or professional, or the professional might have on the desk as they consult. This might be the document parents refer to as they leave the consultant with the diagnosis of 'autism' ringing in their ears.

Whoever applies themselves to the field of study which is Autism Spectrum Disorder will soon become all too aware of the broad scope of the difficulties associated with this condition. Indeed most 'experts' will readily agree that the true scope and nature of this condition is not yet completely understood. Thus it is not surprising that there can exist such a state of contradiction and confusion in the various approaches to ASD, as each researcher views ASD through the lenses of their own philosophical background, and each describes that portion of the truth they have uncovered as best they can using their own particular terminologies.

In the past decade there has been a great amount of activity in the arenas of research and theory development relating to ASD. A newcomer to this field – whether parent or professional - is easily bewildered by the host of new terms and treatment options available.

In the compilation of this directory, the chief aim was to be factual, and then to be brief and clear. Where possible, the approaches have been described in the words of their own proposers or authors. Since it must be understood that the full complexity and scope of each approach could not be covered while still keeping it brief, readers are given the most up-to-date website references possible to encourage further in-depth investigation.

Developments in the study of ASD occur so rapidly that even during the few months it took to complete this work several new approaches had come to the notice of the compiler and were included. It is likely that as it reaches the reader this directory will already be needing an update. It is the compiler's intention to regularly update this work, possibly every year or two.

The reader will find blank pages to receive their own notes as they add to this resource from their own contacts. There are also year-planners and an events section for recording memorable changes or milestones as they occur, or to keep a running record of interventions and scores of tests e.g. the ATEC.

It is my hope that this directory will encourage the reader to continue enquiring, and to embrace change until we have obtained a solution for this condition .... It is expected of professionals that they should continue to refine and perfect their skills and knowledge in service provision to their clients, children or pupils who put their trust in the 'expertise' of each professional with whom they engage.

I also hope that this directory contributes towards clarification and ease of access to information without further cluttering the landscape.

Rosalie Seymour,
Waterford. 2005

TABLE OF CONTENTS

Notes

Personalise with your own notes and contacts

ALTERNATIVE AND AUGMENTATIVE COMMUNICATION AAC

An approach to communication, used when a person is unable to speak, or is unintelligible. It refers to any system that is put in place to enable the speaker or user to interface / communicate with others in his environment. Typically, some visual system is used, e.g. pictures, photographs, line drawings, and spelling systems. These systems may be high-tech, such as computer-assisted communication, or low-tech such as alphabet boards. Clients may use a variety of movements to activate the device, e.g. eye-gaze, manual or head-control; whichever gives the user most control.

www.augcominc.com

APPLIED BEHAVIOUR ANALYSIS – ABA

Based on the theory of operant conditioning (BF Skinner) in which behaviour is reduced to observable and manipulable elements. The focus is on stimulus and response, and the establishment of desirable new behaviour is a result of appropriate reinforcement, and undesirable behaviours are eliminated through a process of extinction (non-reinforcement). The approach was first applied to training children with autism by Dr Ivar Lovaas, and is best known as the Young Autism Project of 1974, UCLA. The approach is outlined in *Teaching Developmentally Delayed Children – The Me Book*, by Dr I O Lovaas.

This approach typically uses careful description, measurement, charts and statistics to determine progress. There are many related approaches and variations of this approach. See:- Precision Teaching, CABAS, TLA, PEAT, IABA

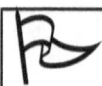

The Geneva Centre

The Geneva Centre for Autism in Toronto, Canada, serves as an information and training centre for professionals and parents to access developments in the field of autistic spectrum disorders.

An excellent source and resource for materials relating to every aspect of enquiry relating to autism. Excellent conferences are held every two years.

www.autism.net/

READ ABOUT

THE FLORANCE SYNDROME

- MAVERICK MINDS :

www.drflorance.com

READ

The Centre for Autism

Website

www.autism.com

AUDITORY INTEGRATION TRAINING – AIT
THE BÉRARD METHOD

An auditory training approach that uses modified music played through earphones to the listener. The music is electronically modulated to alter the sound in such a way that it becomes 'auditory exercise', impacting listening skills at a pre-perceptual, pre-cognitive level. It effectively re-trains the way the ear manages sound. Developed by Dr Guy Bérard, a French Ear-Nose-and Throat specialist who had been working with Dr Alfred de Tomatis (*see Electronic Ear*). Dr Bérard changed the system to more energetic, auditory aerobics. AIT is applied for two half-hour sessions in a period of approximately ten days, using a device called the Audiokinetron , BGC, or Earducator. The effects develop fully after AIT for four months. There is a sound research base supporting the anecdotal reports of benefit.

(see www.sait.org).

Certification :- By Bérard-approved Trainers, internationally. Training : 5 days with examination for competence.

www.georgianainstitute.org

www.aitinstitute.org

BEFRIENDING – NAS, UK

Volunteer befrienders spend a few hours regularly with a family who have a child with ASD (aged 5 to 13). Befrienders can help the child and the family feel less isolated. Befrienders are trained, and reimbursed for out-of-pocket expenses.

www.nas.org.uk

BEHAVIOUR MODIFICATION

The *modification of behaviour* is the goal of all parents, teachers, resource teachers and tutors, therapists of all backgrounds, as well as specialists in behaviour, e.g. psychologists.

Learning is a behaviour, and so are acts of speech, thought, and relating. In this context, a variety of intervention approaches including teaching, therapy, training, would fall under this umbrella term.

However, this term usually refers to the *behaviourist approach* to the management of challenging behaviours. ABA would be a commonly-used behaviourist intervention for autism, as are the ABC (Antecedant Behaviour-Consequence) analysis, Functional Analysis, BIA, and others included in this document. Skills in this area are typically gained by course attendance, seminars and workshops, as well as formal courses in behaviour management.

BIA
THE BEHAVIOURAL INTERVENTION ASSOCIATION
CALIFORNIA

Provide individualised home / community-based programs, consulting, and training workshops that focus on development and implementation of intervention plans for young children diagnosed with autism. Services are recognised by the professional community, in the USA, UK and Ireland. An intervention philosophy that emphasises intensive, individualised curriculum, combining skill-based methodologies. Includes strategies to foster play skills through object focused play to advance communication and social skills.

www.bia4autism.org

BLISS SYMBOLICS

Devised as a symbol system to facilitate global communication, it is employed for users of AAC, i.e non-verbal communicators, who are unable to master literacy, e.g. those with a learning disability. It is more abstract than PCS or Makaton, and therefore allows more flexibility of language and vocabulary e.g. making up new words, and abstract representations. Blissymbolics are used on a variety of computers and synthetic speech devices for communication and literacy learning purposes. Training in its use is done through workshops and publications.

Contact:: Blissymbolics Communications International, Toronto, Canada.

Web: home.istar.ca/~bci

BRAIN DYNAMICS

Originally referred to in the USA as Educational Therapy, or *the Discovery Programme*, and is applied to children (and adults) with specific learning disabilities (dyslexia-type), including high-functioning autism and asperger syndrome, and ADD / H. This approach originated in the work of Dr Wechsler, Dr. Silver, Dr R Hagin, Dr S Orton, Dr A Gallaburda, and others. It acts on the principles of neural plasticity and neuro-cognitive reconstruction.. It is a composite of 27 techniques which are applied in an intensive two-year programme, or longer. It is a language-based approach, establishing linguistic / verbal control of cognition. Admission criteria for professional training: Teachers with three years' experience, or a speech therapy or occupational therapy qualification. Admission criteria for parent training – as help for their own child only.

CONTACTS:- synapseireland@eircom.net

	Notes

Personalise with your own notes and contacts

BRAIN GYM

(*SEE* EDUCATIONAL KINESIOLOGY)

BRAIN SOLUTIONS

Formerly of St Briavels Institute, Wales, Mike and Helen Downey continue their whole-person neuro-developmental approach combining cognitive, metabolic, motor and personal skills development. Parents are trained to provide intensive home-based therapeutic activities, with periodic updates by consultation. This service is provided in many European countries and Kwa-Zulu Natal, Africa.

e-mail: mikehelen@downey6.freeserve.co.uk
tel: 00 44 1594 530287

CARBONE, DR. VINCENT J

Behavioural Analyst who provides consultation, seminars, and mentoring in instructional methods for autism. Emphasis on verbal behaviour.

www.drcarbone.net

CRANIO-SACRAL THERAPY

Sought by many parents of children with autism, this therapy involves gentle manual easing of the flow of the cerebro-spinal fluid as it expresses its rhythmic pulse. Problems with this flow are thought to result in loss of vitality, sleep and mood disorders, and attention deficits.

www.sosnahaingeal.com/Cranio-Sacralinfo.htm

Notes

Personalise with your own notes and contacts

DERBYSHIRE LANGUAGE SYSTEM –DLS

The DLS is an intervention for language that targets early language skills. It is highly structured and carefully graded with objectives that range from single words to long complex sentences, in receptive and expressive forms. The user, whether therapist or teacher, has an assessment tool with which to determine the current levels of skill. These are linked to teaching activities. Course information on enquiry. Workshops last 2 to 3 days in Eire and the UK.

Contacts (Eire) Anne Geraghty, IASLT; Trina Corry (WHB), Imogen Hawes (St Michaels House)

www.derbyshire-language-scheme.co.uk

DEVELOPMENTAL OPTOMETRY

A developmental approach to vision, evaluating not only simple depth of focus, but saccadics, teaming of the eyes, tracking, midline crossing, accommodation speed, and the level of integration of these above. It describes the development of the visual system as part of the motor system. Assessment and therapy measures, observes, and is designed to develop, improve and enhance visual performance to raise levels of performance which in turn affects behaviour and influences how one performs in social, academic, and vocational surroundings. There are many variations of visual therapy, e.g. Visual Management Therapy, Directive Yoked Prisms...

Contacts: College of Optometrists in Vision Development ; info@covd.org ;

Neuro-Optometric Rehabilitation Association International

DIGITAL AUDITORY AEROBICS- DAA

Developed from the Bérard Auditory Integration Training approach, but uses a device other than the SAIT – approved devices. Adheres to the Bérard protocol, delivers the same kind of sound, based on the same principles, and same method of application. Research is under way.

No training required to purchase DAA device, self-study of the manual. Some professionals attend training by Bérard AIT trainer.

Certification – (only if trained by Bérard AIT trainer.)

Contacts:- Stehli, www.georgianainstitute.org

Deana Page, Ennis, Co.Clare 065 6823501

DIRECTIVE YOKED PRISMS

Employed by Dr Mel Kaplan O.D., Tarrytown, New Jersey, who treats children with autism in his practice.. A form of Developmental Optometry, using lenses and visual management training, impacting on the visual processing problems that underlie social and attentional problems, poor eye contact, toe-walking, visual stimulatory behaviours.

Featured in *Dancing in the Rain* – Stehli; and *Rickie* – F. Flach, Research paper:- Ch. Psych.& Human Dev., Vol 27,winter, 1996. Certification: Additional specialisation for optometrists.

Contacts:- The Centre for Visual Management, 150 White Plains Road, Suite 410, Tarrytown, New York, 10591.

DYNAMIC ASSESSMENT

Dr David Tsuriel devised this assessment protocol based on the Learning Potential Assessment Device of Dr Reuven Feuerstein. The tester's role is to 'mediate' concepts during learning, after which the concepts are elicited to gauge the learner's propensity for change. Intelligence is not viewed as static, nor as ranging along a 'bell-curve', and testing is not standardised but dynamic.

www.lab.brown.edu/eac/sped_dynass.shtml

EARLY BIRD PROGRAMME - N.A.S,. UK

A program of workshops, home visits and video training designed to teach parents how best to support their young children newly-diagnosed with autism. Parents attend a three-hour weekly training course for three months, acquiring skills to improve communication and behaviour. It is found to relieve parental stress and build parent partnerships.

www.nas.org.uk

EASE-DISC – MUELLER

An early variation of Bérard AIT, developed at first for people who found that the symptom of painful hearing did not abate after the first course of AIT. .A collection of sound recordings that are played at home on a walkman or hi-fi system through headphones for varying periods of time.

Not approved by Dr Bérard nor IABP, not backed by research.

	Notes

Personalise with your own notes and contacts

EDUCATIONAL KINESIOLOGY – EDU-K / BRAIN GYM

An approach to cognitive development based on the concept of the release of energy for brain-body integration. Developed by Drs Carla Hannaford, Gail and Paul Dennison.

Brain Gym© is the core programme of physical activities that enhance learning ability. It is used by adults, children and seniors to bring about improvements in concentration, memory, reading, organisation skills, language and number skills, speaking and athletic performance. Training is open to all applicants, at varying levels, from introductory basic to professional.

www.braingym.org/

FACILITATED COMMUNICATION

Developed as an approach to alternative and augmentative communication (AAC) in Australia by Rosemary Crossley (DEAL). Further elaborated by Dr. Douglas Biklen at Syracuse University. First used with cerebral palsy, applied to non-verbal people with Autism and Downs' Syndrome. Uses facilitating touch to overcome movement disorder that impedes access to communication aids, e.g. typing devices or letter-boards. Alternately upheld and refuted in court cases, but found useful for encouraging AAC use, and on occasion revealing unexpected literacy in non-verbal people. Not backed by research, yet many documented instances of successful communication through FC, e.g.

'Child of Eternity' – Jorde ; *'Lucy's Story'* – Lucy Blackwell; *'Dancing in the Rain'* – Stehli;

Contacts :- Facilitated Communication Institute, Syracuse, NY; DEAL Communication Centre, AUS

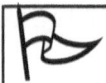

Read:

Advice for Parents of Young Autistic Children,

By Adams, Edelson, Grandin, and Rimland

www.autismwebsite.com/ari/specialinterest/
adviceforparents.html

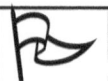

Be sure to look at the

Autism Research Institute

www.autismwebsite.com/ari

Brad's Resource List

In the site for the

Autism Society of Collin County

Is a monster website resource on autism.

Look it up at

http://autism-ascc.org/

FAST FORWORD

CD-ROM and internet-based program to help children build listening and oral language skills. From the work of Merzenich, Tallal, Miller and Jenkins or brain response to sound, and brain plasticity. Uses computer-altered sound manipulation in an adaptive training programme. Found to quickly enhance phonological awareness, processing speed, memory, syntax, sequencing skills, etc. Products are obtained from Scientific Learning$_{TM}$ A range of programs. Used in schools and clinics. Approximately $2000 per client for six-week module. Practitioners train on-line or in workshop attendance.

www.scientificlearning.com

FEUERSTEIN INSTRUMENTAL ENRICHMENT

Dr Reuven Feuerstein developed concepts and interventions such as Mediated Learning Experience, Structural Cognitive Modifiability, and the Learning Potential Assessment Device, and Instrumental Enrichment (IE) Through IE an individual can enhance cognitive integration by means of a series of graded instruments (exercises). A variety of complex cognitive tasks are practised to a level of skill with the intervention of a mediator.

www.icelp.org   www.zipcon.net/~highroad/ie

FLOOR TIME – GREENSPAN APPROACH

The Developmental, Individual-difference, Relationship (DIR) Model Assessment, and Intervention for development and emotional disorders, autism, regulatory disorders involving attention and learning, cognitive, language, motor and sensory problems. Some workshops presented in Ireland: contact   trainingwaysgalway@eirc om.net Training by Stanley Greenspan and Serena Wieder.

www.stanleygreenspan.com

GIANT STEPS

An educational approach to children with autism and Rett's syndrome. An inclusive and successful educational-therapeutic model devised by Darlene Berringer in Montreal, Canada, in 1981. Admits children from 2 yrs of age. With a philosophy of interrelated approaches combining structured education with nutritional therapy, sensory integration, AIT, movement therapies, vision therapy, music and drama. Won the Silver Medal of Canada. Satellites in USA, America, Dubai, Tokyo, London, Paris and Tel Aviv.

www.giantstepsmontreal.com

GROWING MINDS

A programme that balances the child's need for social development with the need to acquire skills and academic competence. Combining ABA with the Option approach. Steve Wertz presents in the UK.

www.autism-programs.com

HANDLE

Founded by Dr Judith Bluestone. Approach to identifying and treating neurodevelopmental disorders for all age clients, including autism. Combines principles from medicine, rehabilitation, psychology, education and nutrition. Based in the USA with branches internationally.

www.handle.org

HANEN

An approach to assessment and development of child communication.

Organised from Toronto, to help young children with or at-risk for language delays communicate to the best of their abilities. There are different levels of training, with resources for parents, Speech Therapists, educators and child carers and community professionals. Backed By Dr B Prizant.. User-friendly materials, providing sound guidelines for assisting children develop their language and communication skills.

www.hanen.org

HEMI-SYNC THERAPY

A brain organisation technique using music to induce particular states of brain-wave activity with multi-layered patterns of sound frequencies. Listened to through headphones, the brain responds by producing a binaural beat that encourages the desired brain activity.

www.hemi-sync.com

HIGASHI - DAILY LIFE THERAPY

Higashi is an outward-bound education system originating in Japan, that emphasises vigorous physical exertion and structured daily routines and the arts. Dr Kiyo Kitahara successfully admitted children with autism who were found to thrive in this system. The Boston Higashi school opened in 1987. .... The programme promotes self-care, and social independence. An evaluation revealed that 50% went to regular employment, 35% to sheltered employment, and 12% went to colleges and universities.

www.mushashino-higashi.org/autism.htm

www.mushashino-higashi.org/ondon.htm

	Notes

Personalise with your own notes and contacts

HOLDING THERAPY / HOLDING TIME

Also known as Direct Synchronous Bonding or Attachment Therapy. Dr Martha G. Welsh, a psychiatrist, used 'forced holding' to repair a range of developmental dysregulatory disorders and severe conduct disorders e.g. arson, ...and found it helpful for some people with autism. This is performed by the parent with the support and guidance of a trained professional. Is believed by some (Dr. Temple Grandin) to be effective due to the deep pressure given – that it acts a form of sensory integration therapy.

www.marthawelch.com

IABA

The Institute for Applied Behaviour Analysis, California, (Dr Gary LaVigna and Dr Thomas Willis). Provide courses for dealing with people with challenging behaviour. Provide non-aversive guidelines and support, positive programming, behaviour assessment, and emergency management

www.iaba.com

INTENSIVE INTERACTION

Developed from the theory of Gary Ephraim who argues for language and social skills learning in a naturalistic setting. A practical approach to interacting with people with a learning disability who have difficulty with social skills and communication. The carer / worker becomes a better communicative partner thus supporting the person with learning disability develop confidence and competence. Is playful and respectful.

www.bild.org.uk

✏️	Notes

Personalise with your own notes and contacts

INTERACT CENTRE

The interact college is a grade 1 specialist day college , with a programme specially developed for older pupils with autism, most pupils being older than 19 yrs. It provides a curriculum for social, communicative, and relational skills, as well as an understanding about autism and how their autism affects the way others see them. All students gain skills for everyday living and pre-vocational skills.

www.theinteractcentre.com

INTERACTIVE METRONOME

A computerised version of the metronome used in music teaching, applied to improving timing and rhythmicity. Acts on the belief that these two functions are basic to the central nervous system, and play an important role in motor planning, sequencing and cognitive functions such as attention and academic achievement.

www.interactivemetronome.com

IRISH SIGN LANGUAGE

Only recently accepted as a language, ISL is promoted by the Deaf community for inclusion in the linguistic experience and education of Deaf students. A Centre for Deaf Studies has been established at Trinity College, Dublin.

IRLEN LENSES – SCOTOPIC SENSITIVITY SYNDROME

Helen Irlen, USA, found that some people have visual systems that react unfavourably to certain bands of the colour spectrum, causing visual perceptual problems.

Irlen discovered the use of colour as a treatment to eliminate perceptual distortions. Treatment may involve wearing coloured lenses specifically suited to the individual, or using colouredoverlays on reading material. Her book *Reading By The Colors (Penguin Putnam)* explains. Applicants for training must have a teaching degree or graduate qualification.

Contact : maritamcgeady@hotmail.com Tel: 01 6280398

www.irlen.com/

JOHANSEN SOUND THERAPY

A variation of Tomatis Electronic Ear therapy, developed in Denmark by Dr Kjeld Johansen. Requires listening to a series of specially recorded music tapes of 10 to 15 minutes duration, daily for 9 months in most cases, but the duration varies according to client needs.

LAMH SIGN SYSTEM

A simplified sign system used in Ireland since 1982 as a standardised introductory communication system for people with learning difficulties.

Training is offered to parents and teachers in a group format, led by certificated trainers. Information on Tutors courses available on request from:

Lamh development officer 051 845454

MAKATON

A sign and symbol language programme for teaching functional communication , language and literacy skills to children and adults with communication difficulties and learning disabilities, through the use of signs and symbols with speech.

www.inclusive.co.uk

www.makaton.org.uk

MARTE MEO

Maria Aarts (Netherlands) developed a technique of assessing and advising communication, particularly in families where a child might have developmental difficulties or behaviour challenges. A family situation is videotaped, typically a mealtime or some other, and this is viewed and communicative moments are discussed, evaluated, and suggestions for change are tabled. It is non-prescriptive, relying on the gaining of insight by the parents. Certification: Maria Aarts will screen any applications to determine suitability, or contact:-

Ireland – martemeo@eircom.net

METAPHON

Howell and Dean advocated direct phonological therapy, based in natural phonology, in a facilitating social context (play), arranged into highly predictable routines to reduce cognitive load. Metaphon Resource Pak 3 elements are screening, process probing and monitoring procedure. The ensuingintervention is systematic and focuses on patterns rather than individual sounds. Play is with toys that exemplify the concept e.g. long vs. short. First stage is phonological process awareness, the second stage is production practise.

Contact :- clothranicholmain@tcd.ie

Notes

Personalise with your own notes and contacts

MEDIATED LEARNING

Occurs when a committed adult / mediator places himself between the child and the learning situation, and guides the child's thought processes. It is the quality of the interaction between the child and adult that establishes building blocks for thinking. As the children are taught thinking processes and strategies, they become active, independent learners. Originally developed as an intervention philosophy and strategy by Dr. Rueven Feuerstein, Israel. He defined the concepts of Structural Cognitive Modifiability by the Mediated Learning Experience. The teaching approach is also known as Instrumental Enrichment. Certification: information available on websites

www.tcml.net www.icelp.org   Contact: Rosens@netvision.net.il

MILLER METHOD

For children with autism spectrum disorders and severe learning disability, situated in Boston, USA. Provide a diagnostic survey, a Miller Umwelt Assessment, parent-child training, and oversight programme, and a summer programme. Distance consultations are also offered.

www.millermethod.org

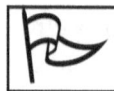
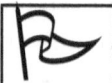
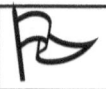

MONTESSORI

Not an academic teaching method, but by encouraging a child to explore and 'research' his environment the child will learn what they need to know to develop knowledge and skills according to their own style. At all ages they experience two three-hour work periods, during which they are not distracted by compulsory breaks or classes, they are allowed to focus and make progress in topics of their own choice, facilitated by a highly-trained adult.

www.montessori.com   www.montessori.edu

M.O.R.E. / SSB

Motor, Oral Respiratory and Eye function, also referred to as Suck-Swallow-Breathe : Devised by occupational therapists Oetter, Richter and Frick for the regulation of attention and for self-regulation. Their manual is explanatory, with many practical guidelines included. Further adapted by Olwen Pate to focus on the fine-motor co-ordinations required for speech production (C.O.R.A.)

Contacts:- www.sensoryintegration.org.uk

MORE THAN WORDS

Adaptation of Hanen for children with autism

MUSIC THERAPY

Music Therapists use music and music interaction to support people with medical, emotional, physical and psychological problems, and may work in health, residential or educational settings. The two-year full-time MA music therapy course is the only course in Ireland leading to a professional qualification in music therapy. Students are admitted from a variety of health and music backgrounds, after a selection process.

www.ul.ie/~iwmc/programmes/mamt/index.html

e-mail: Ellen.Byrne@ul.ie

NEURO-DEVELOPMENTAL DELAY – NDD

Neuro-Developmental immaturity describes the arrest of one or more motor developmental stages which can affect the child's later performance in motor control, eye/hand co-ordination and learning and perceptual skills. NDD therapists see children after the age of 8 years , when they will assess the child and devise movement programmes to remediate or strengthen problem areas. As postural control improves, respiratory control and oral-motor function improve with direct effect on speech production.

www.ndt-ireland.com/ndt_ondon_therapists.htm
inpp@virtual-chester.com

NEURO-DEVELOPMENTAL THERAPY – NDT

Uses knowledge of the nervous system, motor control and sensory systems to improve movement in and for function. Based on the work of Bertha and Karl Bobath, UK, Was primarily applied to cerebral palsy, now applied to a variety of developmental disorders. Training physiotherapists, occupational therapists and speech therapists in an 8-week full-time course.

Bobath Centre London.../   NDTA (USA)

NEURO – COGNITIVE MOBILISATION – NCM

A whole-body approach to language disorders and autism that includes the neurobiological problems, sensory differences and movement disorders, attentional and behaviour problems of these children as the fundamentals for the remediation of communication in all its aspects. Taught to parents, carers and professionals by arrangement, with subsequent supervision and updates. Duration- usually three to four days with upgrades and supervision thereafter.

Contact:: ncm4kids@eircom.net

NEURO-COGNITIVE RECONSTRUCTIVE THERAPY

see **Brain Dynamics**

NEURO-RESPIRATORY THERAPY: ADVANCE

NRT addresses deep core weaknesses within the biomechanics of the respiratory system which affects structure, metabolism, motor skills and cognition. It targets the restoration of normal breathing. Advance is a teaching institute which parents attend with their children, and continue the method at home for 2-3 hours a day for five days a week.

Certification: Bradford University, Health Sciences Dept. Duration: 3 yrs

OSMR – ORAL SENSORY MOTOR RESPIRATORY

Applying the knowledge of motor control and sensory integration to establish motor plans for the range of oral-motor functions required for speech. Focuses on graded control of respiration voicing and oral fine-motor control. Utilises structured oral stimulation and voicing, experiences with a variety of food textures, plus sucking swallowing and blowing fun activities. Taught in three-day seminar / workshop formats, by arrangement. Certification: through course attendance

Contact: rinavanderwalt@hotmail.com

There's a huge amount of speech-related

material on the website of

Caroline Bowen

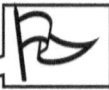

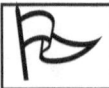

MAPLIN ELECTRONICS
(access them on the 'net)
Has a low-cost sound enhancer
Useful for structured listening etc....

The Mega-Ear Hearing Enhancer

PATTERNING

Developed by Glen Doman and Carl Delacato, and referred to as the Doman-Delacato technique at The Institutes for the Achievement of Human Potential, Philadelphia. Based on the premise that the motor patterns of development precede and form the essential bases for the development of higher cortical functions, including language. The treatment targets the proper development of these early developmental stages, through intensive movement patterns. Parents are typically given home programmes that are reviewed quarterly or more often by arrangement.

www.iahp.org   The Handle Institute. www.handle.org

Institute for Neuro-Physiological Psychology

PEAT
PARENTS EDUCATION AS AUTISM TEACHERS

see Precision Teaching

PECS – PICTURE EXCHANGE SYSTEM

The Pyramid Education System developed a Picture Exchange Communication System – an AAC approach encouraging people with autism and other communication difficulties to initiate communication. Initiation of communication through the exchange of a picture for the desired object while being careful to avoid verbal prompts encourages spontaneity and avoids prompt-dependence. Certification: is 2-tiered. Anyone may use the PECS system, but certification assures skills. Levels are: PECS Implementer; PECS Supervisor –Agency ; Individual Supervisor; Supervisors ;- All certification renewed every two years.

www.pecs.org.uk   www.pecs.com

The Autism Treatment Effectivenesss Survey

Has fascinating data :

See the Autism Research Institute website

www.autismwebsite.com/ari

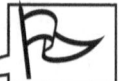

Keep a running progress assessment by using the

ATEC

Autism Treatment Evaluation Checklist

That is scored on the internet

And available for all, free!

www.autismwebsite.com/ari

PLAY THERAPY

Play therapy creates a safe atmosphere where children can express their feelings, explore and learn about social rules and restrictions, and work through their problems. Through their imaginations they can try out different solutions or options. Therapists are trained in the interpretation of play and how to support this exploration. There are several types of play therapy, depending on the psychological school of thought and training of the therapist.

www.play-therapy.com/

PORTAGE

Portage is a home-visiting service for pre-school children with special needs and their families. Originated in Wisconsin, USA. Relies on parental involvement, to develop children play, communication and relationships. Home visitors call weekly , and activities to encourage development are selected with parental input, and parents practice these in-between visits.

www.portage.org.uk

PRECISION TEACHING

A form of ABA as devised by Dr Ken P. Kerr, adding the measurement of speed of response to the drills, believing that increased speed facilitates fluency and generalisation of the learned behaviour. Certification: a variety of courses at various levels are offered.

PEAT :- www.peatni.org

Notes

Personalise with your own notes and contacts

Primary Movement

A movement programme which seeks to inhibit the early fetal reflexes that have persisted abnormally into later developmental stages, and are exerting disruptive influences on postural, motor and cognitive development. Severe persistence of primary reflexes is found in cerebral palsy, although milder persistence is frequently associated with various learning disabilities including dyslexia. A specific movement programme is completed, with effects on motor, visual, emotional and cognitive development.

Training is in two stages, applicants should have experience working with children with learning disabilities.

www.primarymovement.com

Rhythmic Writing

One of the core techniques of Brain Dynamics. Uses large repetitive writing movements coordinated with spoken patterns to enhance neurological organisation and attention. Is a deficit stimulation programme founded on the research into brain plasticity and neuronal re-organisation through motor patterns.

Certification: as in BRAIN DYNAMICS

Samonas Therapy

A variation of Tomatis's Electronic Ear, adapted by Ingo Steinbach.

See   Therapeutic Listening, Tomatis Electronic Ear.

SCERTS
SOCIAL COMMUNICATION EMOTIONAL RELATIONAL AND TRANSACTIONAL SUPPORT

By Dr B Prizant, Dr Amy Weatherby, Rubin, Laurent & Dr P Rydell. A comprehensive multidisciplinary approach for children with autism and their families. To enhance communication and socio-emotional abilities, and to support families. Provide a manual and videotape, introductory workshops. Advanced training to be available once manual is published (2004).

Views the core challenges of autism (ASD) as being social communication and emotional regulation. Focuses on building a child's capacity to communicate using symbolic systems, from pre-verbal to verbal to conversational. Is individualised, family-centred.

www.prizant.com

www.murphyandmurphy.com/barryprizant/

SCOTOPIC SENSITIVITY SYNDROME / SSS

See Irlen Lenses

SENSORY INTEGRATION THERAPY

SI is the neurological process that organises sensation and makes it possible to use the body effectively in its environment. It is the organisation of sensory information for use. SI problems can affect every sensory system.

SI therapy provides carefully sculpted sensory challenges in a structured way through play to stimulate the ordering of the senses, thereby affecting well-being, concentration, communication, and co-ordination. Feeding disorders may have a SI component. Usually performed by SI trained Occupational Therapists and, increasingly, Speech Therapists.

Certification: courses are co-ordinated through Liverpool University. Three week-long modules and an advanced module.

www.sensoryintegration.org.uk

SIBIS: SELF-INJURIOUS BEHAVIOUR INHIBITING SYSTEM

Developed in 1980's by scientists at Johns Hopkins University, consists of a light-weight headgear with a leg or arm-band. Often leads to an immediate, dramatic reduction in self-injurious behaviour, even in cases of violent frequent self-abuse. Research indicates long-term and short-term benefits, including increased socialisation, and placement in less restrictive settings with lessened medication.

www.autcom.org/rights.html

Various reports on SIBIS Research Review International, at www.autismwebsite.com/ari/

SMILE

A therapeutic play approach which encourages language development, enhances interaction and enables children to relate in positive ways with others. Is a home-based programme, with observation and discussion, interactive play activities with video feedback and continued support.

www.autism-smile.co.uk

	Notes

Personalise with your own notes and contacts

SOCIAL STORIES

Carol Gray of Jennison County, USA, devised this method to assist people with autistic ' mind-blindness' to see another person's point of view, and to 'read' social situations. This technique presents acceptable behaviour alternatives in the form of a story which features the client as the chief character.

www.thegraycenter.org/Social_Stories.htm

SON-RISE PROGRAMME ... THE OPTION INSTITUTE

Barry and Samarhia Kaufman used this approach to bring their son, Raun, out of autism. They teach parents of children with a wide variety of challenges, including autism. To enter the world of the child, to scale expectations to the child's level, and learn to relate and interact with the child on their terms, as a fundamental step for encouraging the child to explore beyond the self-imposed restrictions of their condition. Is a very intense 24-hour intervention, in which the child initially remains in one room for all activities. In all activities there is constant accompaniment by an interactive adult trained in this philosophy and method of interaction.

www.son-rise.org

www.optioninstitute.com

SPELL – N.A.S., UK

The NAS clarified a framework of intervention to contain the best-practice elements for autism spectrum disorder. These elements have the following in common: **Strucure **Positive approaches and expectations   **Empathy   **Low arousal   **Links

www.nas.org.uk

Ooops! Wrong Planet syndrome
There is a world of options available in
JYPSY'S SITE…
www/isn.net/~jypsy/

**Once in the site, click on the 'maze' to access the
listings.**

Some Useful Sites for Oral-Motor Stuff

www.pfot.com

www.pdppro.com

www.talktoolstm.com

www.integrate.com

www.speechbin.com

www.superduperinc.com

www.cptoys.com

www.southpawenterprises.com

www.sammonpreston.com

Talk Tools ™ 059 6482869

STRUCTURED LISTENING

The use of personal amplifiers with word lists to highlight consistencies in the language system in order to facilitate the development of active listening and goal-focused imitation. Used for children who have difficulties in mastering the phonological system of the ambient language. Provides the listener with a learning scaffold through word repetition and predictable order.

Contacts: clothranicholmain@tcd.ie

TEACCH

Developed in the early 1980's by Dr Eric Schopler to support behaviour. It centres on the individual's skills, interests and needs. It provides a modified structured teaching environment, typified by schedules (usually visual schedules), and work systems, making expectations clear and explicit. This enables the person with autism to engage their skills independently of direct adult prompting and cueing.. This system can be applied to any teaching environment and the home / residence.

www.teacch.com

THERAPEUTIC LISTENING

A variant of the Tomatis Electronic Ear, presenting a structured program of listening to specially designed music individually selected for each client. It has been integrated into a sensory processing model by Sheila Frick, OTR. It is done as a home program. Also referred to as *Listening with the whole body*.

www.vitallinks.net

www.vitalsounds.com/

TOMATIS ELECTRONIC EAR

Audio-Psycho-Phonology

In the 1950's Dr Alfred Tomatis, A French Ear-Nose-and Throat Specialist developed a radical new approach to listening, persuading that the ear is the foundation of the development of human development, integration, and learning. He proposed that the auditory modality was the key to dyslexia, autism, voice disorders, stuttering, and the majority of oral-verbal linguistic developmental disorders. He devised a sound-stimulation technique involving the use of filtered music (usually Mozart), Gregorian chant, and mother's voice, played through headphones with a bone-vibrator added, for 100 hours in a period of three weeks. Practitioners operate under license to him.

www.tomatis.net

www.tomatis.org/English/

TRAINING IN LEARNING APTITUDE

A form of responsiveness training first developed at the USA Institute for the Deaf, as an entry-level approach to shape attention, eye-contact and imitation skills for children who were deaf. Found to be effective for children with severe language impairment with restricted attention spans and learning skills, and thus applicable to children with autism. Similar to ABA approaches, but less emphasis on statistics and 'discrete trial analysis' that typifies ABA. Taught on application to parents, tutors and related carers.

Contacts: ncm4kids@eircom.net

VERBAL BEHAVIOUR

www.poac.net

Also see *VINCENT CARBONE*

Please Note:
Any oversight is not intended. With the wealth of options available it is inevitable although regrettable that oversights would occur. The compiler would be grateful to receive contributions for inclusion in updates. Please make your contributions in similar concise form to

rseymour@eircom.net

	Notes

Personalise with your own notes and contacts

NEURO-BIOLOGICAL ISSUES AND INTERVENTIONS

DISCLAIMER

PLEASE NOTE THAT THE INFORMATION CONTAINED IN THIS SECTION REPRESENTS THE MOST SUPERFICIAL SUMMARY ONLY OF THESE TOPICS, AND IS IN NO WAY INTENDED AS ADVICE OR RECOMMENDATION . THE AUTHOR CANNOT BE HELD RESPONSIBLE FOR ANY ACTION TAKEN BY ANY PERSON AS A RESULT OF READING THIS INFORMATION . READERS ARE URGED TO NOTE THAT ANY NEUROBIOLOGICAL INTERVENTION SHOULD BE ATTEMPTED ONLY UNDER THE SUPERVISION OF A SUITABLY INFORMED MEDICAL PRACTITIONER.

ALSO NOTE

THAT FOODS MUST NOT BE REMOVED FROM ANY DIET WITHOUT CAREFUL SUPPLEMENTATION AND THE SUPERVISION OF AN INFORMED MEDICAL PRACTITIONER IN COLLABORATION WITH A SPECIFICALLY TRAINED DAN! PRACTITIONER.

IT IS EXTREMELY IMPORTANT THAT DIETARY CHANGES, INVOLVING THE REMOVING OF FOODS FROM A CHILD'S DIET, MUST ALWAYS BE DONE TOGETHER WITH CAREFUL, INFORMED NUTRITIONAL SUPPLEMENTATION TO ENSURE THAT THE CHILDREN DO NOT SUFFER FURTHER EFFECTS OF MALNUTRITION ... GET HELP FROM YOUR DIETITIAN, DOCTOR, OR PAEDIATRICIAN - ASK THEM WHETHER THEY FOLLOW THE DAN! PROTOCOL

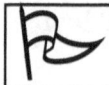

Another Must-Read

**UNDERSTANDING AUTISM:-
THE PHYSIOLOGICAL BASIS AND
BIOMEDICAL INTERVENTION
OPTIONS OF AUTISM SPECTRUM
DISORDERS**
BY
Bryon Jepson

www.cbutah.org

ALLERGY-INDUCED AUTISM
AIA

A UK-based charity dedicated to identifying the underlying causes and biochemical effects of autistic spectrum disorders. Rosemary Kessick is the CEO.

www.autismmedical.com

DR EDWARD DANCZAC

AUTISM MANAGEMENT LIMITED –

While at Manchester Clinic he developed a treatment protocol that he found could be comprehensive and available by tele-conferencing. Provides a detailed parent questionnaire on-line for download.

www.autismmanagement.com/doctor_edward_danczac.htm

BACTERIAL INFESTATION

The presence of mycotoxins from microbacteria in the Gastro-Intestinal tract, such as Clostridia Difficile, can have serious neurotoxic effects that can lead to bizarre behaviours. Testing is via Great Plains Laboratory, the Organic Acids (OAT) and Yeast Combo Sensitivity test.

	Notes

Personalise with your own notes and contacts

CANDIDA CONTROL

Dr William Crooks, and Dr W. Trowbridge, have authored much literature on the implications of candida overgrowth. And its management. Candida is a yeast-like substance present in the gut and elsewhere. In the gut or system of a young child with compromised digestive processes its toxins obstruct many processes, affecting various organ functions including the brain. Candida overgrowth has been implicated in various conditions e.g. M.E. (Yuppie Flu), MS, Alzheimers Disease, and autism.

Testing of organic acids provides a system check for this condition. Management is possible if stringent dietary controls are included, and is usually done in stages over a two-year period, with reported health and neurological benefits.

CHELATION

Is the process whereby a substance is taken which will 'grab' the destructive particle (of the toxic metal such as lead or mercury) and binds tightly with it, pulling it out of the tissue it was embedded in. Then the bonded substance is excreted through the kidneys. Chelation may be done orally or intra-venously. Careful nutritional preparation and supplementation is essential.

NUTRITIONAL RESEARCH INSTITUTE

Dr John McKenna   045897012

www.nrinstitute.net

	Notes

Personalise with your own notes and contacts

COD LIVER OIL

See NUTRITIONAL SUPPLEMENTATION WITH EFA'S

DEFEAT AUTISM NOW! ... DAN!

An initiative of Dr Bernanrd Rimland (Autism Research Institute) who called a symposium of all neurobiologists whose work had application to autism, to compile the first consensus protocol for the neurobiological care of people with autism. Annual conferences are held at which these issues are presented to medical professionals, therapists and parents. Drs Baker and Pangborn published the DAN! Protocol, to guide and advise parents as they request these tests and services form their medical practitioners. Available from most USA autism support groups, and the ARI publications webpage:

www.autism.com/ari

also, see Carin Smit: DAN! Healthcare Practitioner
carinsmit@eircom.net

DIGESTIVE ENZYMES

It appears that the digestive problems of these children can sometimes be overcome or ameliorated through taking oral doses of enzymes. Key nutrients lost through malabsorption may be restored with this support. This measure is to support faulty digestive processes, not to counteract an ongoing poorly managed diet.

DIMETHYLGLYCINE – DMG

A non-toxic metabolite long known as a useful detoxifier and stamina-building product, originating in Russia. Found to boost the immune system, de-stress, and enhance neurological functions e.g. concentration and memory. Beneficial to 50% of people with autism. Dr Bernard Rimland advocates trials of this product before drugs are prescribed. Found useful for clients with drug-resistant seizures. Copious information to be found on DMG and autism, at

www.autism.com/ari

FEINGOLD DIET

In the 1960's D Ben Feingold, Chief of allergy at Kaiser-Permanente Medical Centre, San Francisco, started to use the diet of Dr Lockey of the Mayo clinic, to treat skin conditions and asthma. The finding that by excluding salicylate-containing foods as well as synthetic additives (colourants, preservatives and flavourants) from their diets, the clients' allergy conditions improved alongside their hyperactive and disruptive behaviours led to the further exploration of this link.

www.feingold.org

GLUTEN-FREE / CASEIN-FREE / GLIADIN-FREE DIET

Refers to the neurobiological approach to autism – now more properly includes gliadin – free. Based on the work of Dr Kalle Reichelt (Norway – *see collected net articles*) , the need for this diet is determined by a urine peptide analysis , available from his laboratory in Norway, also at Great Plains Laboratory(USA) and Sunderland Autism Research Unit (UK). The first is generally reported to be more satisfactory. The kits are ordered via e-mail or internet. The sample is prepared by the parents and sent with payment, by courier, with the practitioner's referral note . Results are posted to this practitioner.

It is essential that parents engage a suitably trained and informed professional to advise concerning the dietary changes recommended. Costs for test ; approximately €150 plus courier costs. See DAN! Healthcare Practitioner page 51

www.neurozym.com (Norway)

karlr@ulrik.uio.no

www.gpl4u.com   (USA)

GREAT PLAINS LABORATORY

A comprehensive resource for all manner of neurobiological information and testing. Dr Shaw supervises and advises. A must-read for all parents and professionals of children with ASD and related conditions

www.gpl4u.com

www.greatplainslaboratory.com

GREAT SMOKIES DIAGNOSTIC LABORATORY

Offer a comprehensive digestive stool analysis, and are committed to providing the most valuable up-to-date information about autism and ASD-related issues.

www.gsdl.com/

HAIR MINERAL ANALYSIS
See MINERAL HAIR ANALYSIS

HEAVY METAL TOXICITY

High levels of toxic metals deposited in body tissues and subsequently the brain may cause significant developmental and neurological damage, including autistic symptoms, depression, increased irritability, anxiety, insomnia, hallucinations, memory loss, aggression, and other disorders.

Laboratory testing determines levels of heavy metal deposits. Treatment usually involves removal of the heavy metal source and use of chelating agents.

DR KALLE REICHELT

(Urine Peptide Analysis - Norway)

Requires a sample of first fasting / morning urine. See gluten-free etc. on page 53. These results give essential information for managing the dietary changes. Contact Dr. Reichelt for instructions on testing: karlr@ulrik.uio.no

KETOGENIC DIET

It is found that in some cases, seizure control may be achieved through dietary manipulation, in which carbohydrates are eliminated and proteins and fats increased, producing a state of 'ketosis'. This must be carefully monitored and scrupulously applied by specifically-trained supervisors.

www.epilepsyfoundation.org/answerplace/Medical/treatment/diet

	Notes

Personalise with your own notes and contacts

KIRKMAN LABORATORIES

The only laboratory to have responded to Dr Bernanrd Rimland's original call for tenders to produce a vitamin / mineral supplement specifically suited to children with autism. Also developers of other non-allergenic nutritional supports.

www.kirkmanlabs.com

L-CARNITINE

Is an energy modulating nutrient that enables EFA's to be metabolised as fuel. It is Important to use only pure L-carnitine, not the one buffered with salts (fumerate / tartrate). Used for stroke victims, Alzheimers patients, and autism.

MINERAL HAIR ANALYSIS

It is thought by many that the analysis of the hair provides a long-term indicator of the status of the body's mineralisation. E.g. the history of toxicity over a three-month period, that is less affected by what was had for the last meal as is the case in blood-work. This offers a less traumatic testing alternative for some investigations, than the drawing of blood from a child with autism.   Request information from Yvette Busch at   service@microtrace.de

✏️	Notes

Personalise with your own notes and contacts

NUTRITIONAL SUPPLEMENTATION
WITH ESSENTIAL FATTY ACIDS (EFA)

Medical research indicates the possibility that fatty acid deficiencies are found in two-thirds of children with ASD and related conditions. Parents report improvements in behaviour, attention, sleep, and behaviours such as speech when children supplement with these nutrients.

www.autism.about.com article *Essential Fatty Acids*

ORGANIC ACID TESTING

The testing of urine for the status of the organic acids gives invaluable information regarding the presence of the gastro-intestinal micro-organisms, e.g. that might be responsible for disbiosis with negative effects on health and brain function. Some laboratories offer an organic acids and yeast combo sensitivity all-in-one test.(e.g. Great Plains Laboratory)

SECRETIN

Secretin is a natural substance produced by all mammals, and is neither a drug nor harmful. Its use is controlled in the USA by the FDA for the diagnosis of gastrointestinal problems. A parent of an autistic child, Victoria Beck, reported that after such an investigation, her son's autism disappeared for a while, and did so each time the substance was administered. Many trials later, at present the secretin of porcine origin is no longer available, and the synthetic secretin might not be as effective, although studies continue to report improved GI function, with increased socialisation (including language) in a subset of children who are anti-gliadin IgG positive and have low secretin values.

http://autism.com/ari/specialinterest/secretin.html

SULFATION

Dr Robert Sinaiko (USA) and Dr Rosemary Waring (UK) demonstrated that many children with diagnoses ranging from autism to hyperactivity are unable to detoxify from phenolic compounds due to insufficiency of the enzyme pheno-sulfo-transferase – PST. They describe the test to identify this problem, and interventions to assist this metabolic process.

SUNDERLAND – DR PAUL SHATTOCK - (THE AUTISM RESEARCH UNIT)

A well-known laboratory for the investigation of the gastro-intestinal problems of children / adults with autism.

http://osiris.sunderland.ac.uk/autism/

SUPER-NU THERA

A super-nutrition combination designed by Dr Rimland and produced by Kirkman Laboratories, to provide a spectrum of vitamins and minerals with no colourant, flavourant or filler, thus useful for people with autism . Particularly rich in vit B_6.

www.kirkmanlabs.com

Trimethylglycine – TMG

The 'big brother' of DMG, it releases an additional methyl (oxygenation) molecule when ingested , to convert harmful homocysteine in the blood to SAMe... which becomes a precursor for seratonin, a neurotransmitter. Having shed the extra methyl, it becomes DMG, providing those known benefits in the system. Particularly beneficial for cardio-vascular problems. Information on the Kirkman website :

www.kirkmanlabs.com

Urocholine

See Mary Megson's article on Natural Vitamin A for information on the use of urocholine.

Ultra-clear Sustain / Ultra-care For Kids

A nutritional supplement produced by PPC Galway, in a rice-base, containing many amino-acids and proposed by some as a nutritional support for the picky eater and those with serious digestive problems. Contains L-glutamine to heal a leaky gut.

Available by prescription from your practitioner.

✎	Notes

Personalise with your own notes and contacts

Glossary Of Terms In Autism And Related Disorders

AAC   See Alternative and Augmentative Communication

ABA   See Applied Behavioural Analysis:

ABC   Aberrant Behaviour Checklist, by Aman & Singh, giving a measurement of the following behaviours:- hyperactivity, lethargy, irritability, abnormal speech, and Stereotypy . Used to measure change due to interventions in autism.

ABR audiometry   Acoustic Brainstem Response audiometry – A method of determining the approximate hearing threshold of a client who cannot respond adequately for behavioural / response audiometry. Reads the brain's response to sounds.

Acquired epileptic aphasia   See Landau-Kleffner Syndrome

ADD   See Attention Deficit Disorder.

ADI   Autism Diagnostic Interview – Developed by the Medical Research Council in London – found to be more precise than the CARS

ADOS   Autism Diagnostic Observation Schedule – developed by Sir Michael Rutter.

AIA   Allergy Induced Autism – a UK-based association exploring the dietary interventions for autism, Chaired by Rosemary Kessick.

AIT   See Auditory Integration Training – the Bérard Method.

Alternative and Augmentative Communication   Any system of symbols that enables a non-verbal person to participate in communication, or make their needs known, or to better understand what is being communicated to them. Not gesture. Usually some visual system, e.g. pictures, letter-board, Bliss symbols, PECS.

ANDI   Autistic Network for Dietary Intervention.

Apraxia   Also known as Developmental Co-ordination Disorder.

Applied Behavioural Analysis   A development from Operant Conditioning in which behaviours are established or extinguished by the application or withholding of reinforcers. Applied to the treatment of autism by Dr I Lovaas (see Young Autism Project, UCLA).

ARI / ARRI   Autism Research Institute – director Dr Bernard Rimland, author of Childhood Autism

Articulation disorder   A speech problem in which the child / adult substitutes speech sounds, sometimes causing problems with unintelligibility of speech.

Asperger's Disorder   Another form of autism as described by Dr Hans Asperger. A term more commonly used to identify high-functioning, usually verbal children with fixations and movement disorders..

ASA   Autism Society of America

ASD   Autistic Spectrum Disorder. Includes all children with autism or autistic-like developmental disorders.

Audiokinetron   The sound modulation system devised by Dr Berard and built by Pierre Suire to provide AIT.

Audiology   The diagnosis of hearing disorders and their treatment including the fitting of hearing aids.

Audiometry   The diagnosis of disorders of hearing through testing response to sounds.

Auditory hyperacusis   An over-sensitivity to increases in the loudness of sound. Can vary from mildly irritating to severely debilitating reaction of the hearing to sounds that would not bother most people. Found in 40% of people with autism, and related disorders.

Auditory integration training   The Berard Method . Using modulated sound to enhance listening skills / auditory processing. (

Not the same as Therapeutic Listening, which links with the Tomatis Method.)

Auditory processing   What the brain does with the sound signal, once it is heard. Is a precursor system to perception.

Auditory processing disorder   Difficulty making full use of the heard auditory signal. Includes difficulties with loudness response / registration, with listening in noise, attending to sounds, with localisation of sound. Underlies many speech- language problems.

Auditory processing speed   The rate of transmission of the auditory signal via the brainstem to the left temporal area of the brain. Slow processing (brainstem transmission time) is found to underlie language-based developmental disorders like dyslexia, autism.

Auditory Verbal Agnosia   Also known as 'word-deafness', the child is unable to comprehend in the auditory channel. Acts as if profoundly deaf but can hear. A feature of Landau-Kleffner Syndrome.

Aversives   A strategy to address challenging behaviours that uses unpleasant consequences for these behaviours to decrease their occurrence. Range from a warning tone of voice, 'no', a head-shake or frown, averted gaze, loss of privileges, through to a loud shout, slap or physical punishment.

Basal ganglia   A structure in the brain, which regulates movement outputs between the motor cortices and the thalamic sensory nuclei, by means of neuro-chemical regulation.

Behaviour modification   Any intervention that seeks to alter the way an individual acts. All therapies are behaviour modification approaches. This term usually refers more specifically to changing conduct. Also includes ABA.

Behavioural audiometry   The testing of hearing by presenting a signal and observing the client's response to it. Usually requiring the client signal registration of the heard sound, e.g. by pressing a button, etc.

Bliss symbolics   A system of simplified symbols for written language and communication for those who cannot use the alphabet.

Brain allergies   An early term to refer to the effect of certain foods in the development of such neurological disorders as autism, attention disorders, aggression and hyperactivity, also mood disorders. Now more properly referred to as Neuro-biological disorders, also food intolerances.

Brain dynamics   An integrated programme of therapeutic techniques targeting Cerebral Dissonance Syndrome. It is a deficit stimulation programme using language to provoke higher levels of neuro-integration. Of application for normal learners and developmental disorders. Establishes language dominance in the left hemisphere (where it should be).

Brain gym   Originating from the work by Paul Dennison and Carla Hannaford, applying kinesiology (integrating movements) to enhance brain functions for learning.

Brain hemispheres   The two halves of the brain, the left and the right cerebral hemispheres.

Brain scan   A neuro-imaging tool by means of which a pictographic representation is given of blood-flow or glucose metabolism, using radio-active isotopes injected into body fluids, as tracers.

Brain stem   The structures between the spinal column and the cerebral hemispheres, including the medulla oblongata, the pons and the midbrain, with the hypothalamus, thalamus, limbic system and basal ganglia.

Brainstem audiometry   See ABR

Canon Communicator   A hand-held typing device that produces a strip of paper with the typed sentences. Keyboard arranged in ABC order, with a dot-matrix printout format. Used as an AAC device.

Candida Albicans A yeast/fungus which lives and proliferates everywhere, but especially in the human intestine, in the absence of friendly bacteria, such as lactobacillus acidophilus.

CARS Childhood Autism Rating Scale – sometimes used as a diagnostic tool for autism.

Casein The protein in mammalian milk, whether cow, goat or human.

(Central) auditory processing See Auditory processing

(Central) auditory processing disorder See Auditory processing disorder.

Cerebellum The part of the brain beneath the hemispheres in the posterior section of the skull, responsible for sensory-motor integration.

Cerebral dissonance syndrome As described by M. Gazzaniga , A. Gallaburda, Rosen and others. A condition of competitive hemispheral dominance for language contributing towards attention deficits, dyslexia, lack of cerebral dominance and lack of dominance, laterality and directionality, as well as other language-based learning deficits.

Cerebral hemispheres See Brain hemispheres.

CHAT Checklist for Autism in Toddlers –used for 18-month-olds, by Baron-Cohen, Allen and Gillberg.

Chelation therapy The removal of toxic heavy metals from the cells of the body through the introduction of a binding agent to 'flush' these toxins from the system. Can be done orally or by intravenous infusion.

Chiropractic manipulation An intervention to release spinal pressure and correct misalignment / sublaxation of joints, particularly the vertebra.

Circumlocution   The tendency to talk around a topic in a vaguely related way without specific content, commonly when the speaker can't recall the specific label for an object or action.

Connors Behaviour Rating Scale   Used to quantify the aberrant behaviours of children with ADD and related disabilities (including autism).

Corpus callosum   The part of the brain that connects the two cerebral hemispheres. It is composed of connecting fibres of brain cells, or 'white matter'

Cranio-sacral therapy   Gentle manual easing of the flow of cerebro-spinal fluid by a suitably qualified therapist.

CSBS   Communication and Social Behaviour Scale, by Wetherby and Prizant,, for early identification of infants who might be at-risk for autism.

DAA   Digital Auditory Aerobics – a variant of Berard Auditory Integration Therapy, in which the pre-recorded modulated music is played to the client through a final modulating stage. Adheres to the Berard protocol of ten days of two sessions per day.

DAN!   Defeat Autism Now! – an initiative by Dr Bernard Rimland of ARI, to combine information on metabolic interventions in autism. Produces the DAN! Protocol, to inform parents of options and guide them in their requests for these tests from their physicians.

Decibels   in audiology - The unit of loudness of sounds.

Developmental co-ordination disorder See Dyspraxia / Apraxia.

Developmental optometry   The assessment and treatment of problems of visual function, beyond convergence and focus testing, including tracking,, eye movements, teaming, and hand-eye co-ordination.

Digestive enzymes   Enzymes are protein molecules that act as catalysts. Digestive enzymes cause the food to be broken down into smaller particles that are nutrients for the body's use.

Directive yoked prisms   A treatment applied to autism by Melvyn Kaplan, New Jersey, for children with visual problems.

Discrete Trial Training   Also known as Discrete Trial Analysis – the technique of behavioural intervention whereby one aspect of behaviour is addressed at a time, with careful control of all other variables. The central technique of ABA.

DMAE   Di-methyl Aminoethanol – used in Chelation therapy

DMG   Di-methylglycine – a non-toxic metabolite used to detoxify and to promote healing,. It also enhances mental functions, due to its oxygenating effect on the blood. Found useful and non-harmful for many people with autism.

Dopamine   A neuro-transmitter regulating movement, attention and tremor.

DPP-IV   Dipeptidyl peptidase –IV, a digestive enzyme shown to be deficient in people with autism. DPPIV is only helpful if casein, gluten is removed from the diet. It will then help to protect the immune system and assist with calcium absorption.

DSM-IV   Diagnostic and Statistical Manual for Mental Disorders, 4th edition, used for diagnosing psychiatric conditions including autism.

Dynamic assessment   Based on the methods of Reuven Feuerstein, the use of the assessment tool to also gauge modifiability of learning styles.

Dysarthria   Defects of articulation which are caused by either central or peripheral nerve damage or impairment.

Dyspraxia   A milder form of Apraxia.

E2   A checklist compiled by Dr Bernard Rimland of the Autism Research Institute, to assess numerically the probability that a child will be diagnosed as autistic or autistic-like. Not of itself a diagnostic instrument, but useful as a part of the process of arriving at a diagnosis. Available to parents free of charge on request.

E3 Included with the E2, an assessment of treatments for autism that parents have tried and their evaluation of the effectiveness of each.

Earducator Sound modulation system devised in South Africa by Rosalie Seymour and built by Tim Hagen to provide Berard AIT.

ECG Electro-Cardio-Gram – testing the electrical heart functions.

Echolalia The usually meaningless repetition of words and phrases by an individual who may have no useful speech of their own.

Educational kinesiology Also known as Brain Gym

EEG Electro-Encephalo-gram – testing electrical brain function.

Electronic ear The sound modulation system devised by Dr Alfred de Tomatis, on which Therapeutic Listening is based.

Essential fatty acids- EFA Fatty acids – a molecule containing carbon, hydrogen and oxygen atoms together which make up building blocks of fats and oils found in the human diet. Linoleic acid and alpha linoleic acid are 'essential' because these fatty acids start the Omega 3 and Omega 6 metabolic pathways, and as such have to be derived from the diet as the body cannot produce them.

Face Blindness Propagnosia – the inability to recognise faces.

Facilitated communication The use of a system of support, usually resistive touch, to enable an AAC user to access the communication board more efficiently. Has been helpful to non-verbal people with autism, and other disorders, who have nonetheless been able to communicate through his approach.

Facilitation Any system / action whereby the execution of a movement is made more efficient . It includes, but is not limited to , facilitating music or rhythm, facilitating touch, facilitating emotional support.

Feingold diet   Dr Ben Feingold demonstrated the beneficial effects of removing sugars, colorants, flavourants and preservatives from the diets of hyperactive children. Foods containing salicylates and high in phenolic compounds are often problematic to these children.

Fine-motor co-ordination   Managing the movements of small-muscle actions smoothly, especially referring to hand, eye and mouth movements.

Floor Time   The Greenspan approach, also called DIR.

Food intolerance   Previously called brain allergies, but not an allergic reaction: the inefficient digestion of certain foods does not produce the required nutrients , but the undigested particles are toxins which interfere with neurological and immuno-functioning.

Food sensitivities   As in food intolerance. Differs from allergies, in that there may be no raised IgA/E/G, but these foods cause physical and mental problems if consumed by the individual.

Fragile X   This syndrome is the most common cause of inherited mental retardation, seen in approximately one in 1,200 males and one in 2,500 females.. DNA testing is done to determine whether the gene mutation has occurred.

Frequency   In audiology - refers to the pitch of the pure-tone sound.

Frontal lobe   The part of the cerebral hemispheres at the forehead, thought to be responsible for the highly-evolved human cognitive attributes, including morality and evaluation.

GARS   Gillingham Autism Rating Scale

Giant steps   A broad-based intervention programme from Montreal, Canada, for children with autism. Has received many awards for the results achieved. Many programmes have been established internationally.

Gliadin   The protein in pulses, including soya, beans, nuts. Found to be problematic for some children with ASD

Gluten   The protein in grains such as wheat, oats, barley and rye.

Grommets   Also P-E tubes or ventilation tubes. Used drain fluids from the middle ear.

Gross motor co-ordination   The co-ordination of large movements, as performed by the whole arm, or leg, or whole body.

Hair analysis   A method to assess for heavy metal toxicity by collecting a sample of recent hair growth for laboratory analysis.

Holters sleep study   A 24-hour EEG, which is done by means of a special EEG machine, to determine changes in brain wave function over prolonged periods of time

Hanen   An approach taught to parents to encourage and support the learning of language by young children.

Healing crisis   The experience of worsening of symptoms after treatment has begun, that might signal the commencement of recovery or improvement as the body's immuno-defences begin to operate more efficiently. Often occur in detoxification programs.

Hearing loss   The loss of acuity / crispness of hearing, as when it takes greater volume for a sound to be just-heard. Varying degrees and types of hearing loss are identified by an audiologist.

Heavy metals   The term heavy metal refers to any metallic chemical element that has a relatively high density and is toxic or poisonous at low concentrations. Examples of heavy metals include mercury (Hg), cadmium (Cd), arsenic (As), chromium (Cr), thallium (Tl), and lead (Pb).

Hemi-sync   An auditory technique using music to set up binaural 'beats' that influence brain waves, to enhance calm states, or attentiveness.

Herxheimer effect   See healing crisis.

Higashi system   Also known as Daily Life Therapy. A Japanese educational system emphasising physical fitness and creativity.

Hippocampus   A portion of the temporal lobe called the hippocampus, regulating both memory and emotion and is part of the limbic system.

Holding Therapy   See Welch Method.

Hyperactivity   A neurological condition resulting in restlessness, whether mental or physical.

Hyperacusis   An auditory processing disorder in which sounds are perceived more loudly than normal. See auditory hyperacusis.

Hyperlexia   Precocious reading ability. Sometimes found in non-verbal children with autism.

Hypo-acusis   Another term for hearing loss.

Hypotonia   See Low muscle tone

IAA   Irish Autism Alliance – chairman Cormack Rennick... An association of the parents of younger autistic children

IAG   Indolyl-Acrolyl-Glutathione

ICD 10   International Classification of Diseases – 10th edition.

IgA   Protein immunoglobulin A (IgA): The IgA protein, an antibody, is a normal part of the body's immune system, the system that protects against disease

IgE   One of five classes of immunoglobulins made by humans (the others being IgA , IgD , IgG and IgM). Main function seems to be to protect the host against invading parasites. However, the same antibody-cell combination is also responsible for typical allergy or immediate hypersensitivity reactions such as hay fever , asthma , hives and anaphylaxis.

IgG   IgG is the most common type of antibody , comprising about 80% of the body's total. It is equally divided between the blood and interstitial fluid. IgG antibodies represent a large vocabulary of antigen recognition molecules.

ISA   Irish Society for Autism, Director Pat Matthews.

I S L   Irish Sign Language

Inborn errors of metabolism   The list includes: defective proteins, defects in carbohydrate metabolism, defects in cholesterol and lipoprotein metabolism, mucopolysaccharide and glycolipid diseases, errors in amino acid and organic acid metabolism, defects in non-amino acid nitrogen metabolism, errors in mitochondrial fatty acid oxidation, defects in nucleotide metabolism, disorders in metal metabolism and transport, disorders of peroxisomes, diseases associated with defective DNA repair mechanisms.

Inner ear infection   An infection of the inner ear; the cochlea, or nerve cells, or vestibular (balance mechanism). See nerve deafness.

Instrumental enrichment   A cognitive re-training method devised by Dr. Reuven Feuerstein by means of which several cognitive stimulation "instruments" (cognitive exercises) were designed to enhance problem solving, strategic thinking, spatial reasoning,, verbalisation and higher level thinking skills in low functioning individuals, by means of a mediator-led process of reciprocal speech.

Interactive metronome   A computerised version of the timing metronome used in music, applied to improve rhythmicity in order to improve attention, motor planning and cognitive functions.

Irlen lenses   See Scotopic Sensitivity Syndrome

IVIG   Intra-venous Immunoglobulin

Johansen therapy   A variant of Tomatis Sound Therapy.

Ketogenic diet   Used to control some resistant epilepsies, through a diet high in fats and low in carbohydrates, so that the body burns fat instead of glucose. Requires careful medical monitoring.

Kinesiology   The study of the muscles in relation to movement and pain relief.

Lamh sign system   A signing system developed in Ireland for use by the learning disabled, with similarities to Makaton.

Landau-Kleffner Syndrome – LKS   A seizure disorder whose only sign might be the rapid / sudden loss of language, comprehension and eye contact, and may often be mistaken for Autism.

Learning Disability   (In Ireland and the UK): mental handicap; (in the USA and elsewhere)- dyslexia, and specific learning disability

Limbic system   The mid-brain system which regulates mood and attitude, it is the centre of the emotions, and affect non-verbal communications. Thought to be key to the storage and retrieval of memories.

Low muscle tone   A neurological condition in which the muscles' resting state of 'residual tone' is too low, resulting in postural instabilities and poor fine-motor co-ordination.

LSR   Least Restrictive Environment.

Lymphatic system   The lymphatic system defends the body from foreign invasion by disease causing agents such as viruses, bacteria, or fungi. The lymphatic system consists of: The bone marrow, spleen, thymus gland, lymph nodes, tonsils, appendix, and a few other organs.

Makaton   A UK system of symbols and signs to facilitate communication by the learning disabled population.

Mediation   Reuven Feuerstein's concept of the process by which the learner interacts with the 'teacher', whose role is to sharpen critical thinking through challenges and open-ended questioning.

Melatonin   A hormone that acts as a neurotransmitter, important in the regulation of sleep patterns (amongst other functions.) Found to be an effective natural help for sleeping problems.

Mentalising   See 'Mind-Blindness'.

Midbrain   Part of the brainstem , it relays messages to and from the brain, cerebellum & spinal cord .

Middle-ear hearing loss   The condition of mechanical obstruction of the passage of sound through the middle-ear, through fluid build-up (infection) or disruption of the bony chain. The resulting hearing loss is usually mild to moderate.

Middle-ear infection   An infected fluid build-up behind the eardrum, that impedes the passage of sound and resulting in some middle-ear hearing loss. It may resolve naturally, or may cause intense pain until pressure is relieved through insertion of grommets or the bursting of the eardrum. Some non-infective fluid build-ups (as during a cold) are erroneously called 'infections'.

Mind-blindness   The theory (UK-based) that the key deficit of autism is the inability to understand another's point of view, or perspective. The ability to do so is believed to be essential to communication and socio-emotional skill.

Mixed laterality / mixed dominance   The profile of having a dominance for the hand on one side, with eye-or foot-dominance on the opposite side. Might indicate inefficient organisation of language dominance in the hemispheres.

MTW – More Than Words   The adaptation of Hanen for autism.

Morphology   The management of tense markings, plurals and other grammatical small words called functors. Comprehension and use of these may be impaired.

Movement disorder   Another term for co-ordination problems, but highlighting the issue of the planning of motor sequences inherent in this problem.

Muscle tone   The degree of tension normally present when the muscles are relaxed or in a resting state.

NAD   Nicotine-Adenine-Dinucleotide, one of the chemical co-factors of the Krebs cycle essential for the production of energy. Can be supplemented orally or intravenously.

NAS National Autism Society – UK.

Neonatal audiometry Usually the assessment of the newborn's startle response to a loud sudden-onset sound. This test is used to screen neonates for profound hearing loss.

Nerve deafness Inner-ear hearing loss – caused by damage or disease of the inner ear, in which the nerve cells may die. An irreversible and usually more profound hearing loss. It may be present from birth, or develop over time as a progressive condition.

Neuro-biological issues The inborn or acquired conditions in which the metabolism cannot adequately manage ingested substances, due to excessive sensitivity, or the inability to adequately rid the system of toxins. The toxic load affects all organs, including the brain, leading to cognitive, mood and behavioural symptoms.

Neuro-cognitive reconstructive therapy Also known as Brain Dynamics – intensive motor- perceptual –cognitive interventions with an oral language base – an effective bridge between NDT / SI and speech therapy to effect classroom and socio-emotional success

Neuro-developmental delay NDD, also called NDT – a movement approach to developmental disorders, originating in physiotherapy for cerebral palsy. NDD practitioners do not treat children under the age of 8 yrs, whereas NDT is applied to infants and all ages.

Neuroleptic Refers to medication to control seizures.

Neuro-transmitters Brain chemicals (of gastric origin) that mediate impulse transmission, either to facilitate or inhibit these.

NLP Neuro-linguistic programming, or can refer to Natural Language Paradigm.

Normal hearing The point of loudness at which the sound signal is 'just heard' – which should range between 0dB and 15dB for children, and 0dB and 25dB for adults.

NOS As in PDD-NOS – 'not otherwise specified', a classification in the DSM IV – a category subject to fierce debate as to its validity.

Nutritional deficiency This term refers to the way in which children may eat adequate amounts of food, but still be nutritionally under-supplied of necessary elements for their particular needs.

Nutritional supplementation The practice of adding specific nutrients to the diet to ensure adequate supply for the unique metabolic needs of the individual.

Nutritional therapy The understanding that the body is able to heal itself, if the correct nutritional environment is created – a careful understanding of inborn errors of metabolism needs to accompany any nutritional therapy.

NVLD Non-Verbal Learning Disability.

Obsessive-Compulsive Disorder One of the most common neuropsychiatric disorders, in which the person must have obsessions, or compulsions, or both.

OCD See Obsessive-Compulsive Disorder

Occipital lobe The posterior part of the brain where visual processing predominates.

ODD Oppositional-Defiant Disorder

Operant conditioning The original term to denote the action of stimulus – response – reinforcement that is the basis of ABA, and behavioural psychology.

Oppositional-defiant disorder- ODD A severe conduct disorder characterised by low levels of compliance.

Optimum nutrition As different from the RDA (recommended daily allowance) of a nutritional element. The RDA is the baseline, minimum requirement of a nutrient, where the optimum level of intake of that nutrient will vary with age and activity.

Optometry   The testing of vision, usually to determine convergence and depth of focus, possibly leading to the prescription of lenses.

Outer ear infection   Also known as Otitis Externa – an infection mainly caused by an effusion from the membrane the lines the outer ear canal.

Painful hearing   Also called Hyper-acusis:- the key symptom is a painful response to sounds that are normally not bothersome to others. Associated with severe emotional reactions, e.g. depression, social withdrawal, and aggression.

Parietal lobe   That part of the cortex sandwiched between the occipital and temporal lobes, mainly involved in the processing of visual-spatial information.

Patterning   The development and utilisation of motor patterns from basic fundamental reflexes, usually referring to Intensive rigorous re-training of neurological control for movement creating new neurological sensory-motor imprints.

PDD   Pervasive Developmental Disorder – in practice, used to denote children with milder forms of autism spectrum disorder, or very young children before the age when they might receive the diagnosis of autism.

PECS   Picture Exchange Communication System

PEP   Parents for Exceptional Progress – USA.

Also refers to Psycho-Educational Profile

PEP-R   Psycho-Educational Profile – Revised: an assessment of the features of the developmental difficulties of autism that highlights areas for intervention.

Peptides   Bits of half-digested proteins found in the bloodstream..

P-E tubes   Grommets, or ventilation tubes, which are inserted into the eardrum to allow the normalisation of air pressure in the middle ear, and the draining of fluid from the middle ear during effusion / infection.

PET scan   Positron-Emission Tomography

Phenolic compounds   Phenols are poisons – toxins, which need to be rendered non-toxic by means of an enzyme called Phenol-sulphur-transferase. Phenols are high in food additives, e.g. flavourants and colourants.

Pheno-sulfer-transferase- PST   The enzyme which attaches a sulphur atom to the phenolic compound in order to allow the excretion of the toxin.

Phonology   The ability to manage contrasting speech sound features and speech sound information.

Phonological-syntactic deficit   These speakers are disfluent, speak in short sentences, and often make morphological errors.

Pragmatic language disorder   Difficulty with the use of language in social contexts.

Precision teaching   The form of ABA taught by Dr Ken Kerr, focusing on speed of response.

Primitive reflexes   These are reflexes that develop during uterine life. They should be fully present at birth and are gradually inhibited by higher centres in the brain during the first 12 to 24 months of life. If activated at a later stage they can interfere with the development of more complex skills.

Proprioperception   The deep-muscle and ligament sense of position of the limbs or body in space. An essential sense for body image and motor co-ordination.

Pure-tone audiometry   Using pure-tones generated by an audiometer to assess hearing threshold.

Purkunje Cells   Cells found in the cerebellum, regulating motor memories and fine motor movements, sensory modulation.

Recruitment   The abnormal response of the inner ear nerve cells to sound, in which a small increase in loudness is perceived as very large.

Response audiometry   A form of auditory testing that requires a repeatable, reliable response from the client.

Reticular Activation System   RAS – That system in the brain which functions to create wakefulness and attention when stimulated and is mainly sub-consciously triggered.

Rett's syndrome   Degenerative condition that mimics autism in its early stages, and is only diagnosed in girls.

Rhythmic writing   One of the key techniques of NCRT or Brain Dynamics.

Samonas   An adaptation of Tomatis Sound therapy.

Savant   Also called autistic-savant.

Scotopic sensitivity syndrome-SSS   Also called Irlen syndrome: a condition of visual perceptual distortion due to certain parts of the colour spectrum, that can be treated through the wearing of such coloured lenses as suit the sufferer.

Secretin   A pancreatic hormone initially used to test digestive processes, but was found to have therapeutic benefits in some children

Self-Stimulatory Behaviour   'stim's'… the repetitive behaviours of children (with or without an autism diagnosis), which provide some sensory input, that may be calming, or an expression of distress, but may also be self-injurious or socially unacceptable.

Semantic disorder   The client has difficulty understanding the meaning of words, especially abstract or multi-meaning words. Idioms are poorly understood. Topic control may be a difficulty due to an inability to identify the keyword of an utterance.

Semantic-Pragmatic Disorder   Fluent, well-formed speech with echolalia in young speakers. Later it is seen as delayed echolalia (long monologues of learned speech, e.g. from video programmes). Verbal comprehension is poor, and literal. Circumlocutions may be evident.

Sensory deprivation   A situation in which there are fewer sensory experiences available to an individual than the minimum needed to maintain optimum functioning. Can occur deliberately (brainwashing technique) or be due to illness. E.g. auditory deprivation due to ear infections, or neonatal incubation.

Sensory diet   (Pat Wilbarger, USA) Sensory experiences placed throughout a person's day, to provide strong integrating sensory experiences to maintain a calm-alert state for optimum functioning.

Sensory integration   The efficient co-ordination of sensory information for the purpose of the successful accomplishment of a task.

Sensory modulation   An internal process: the neurological control of the level of intensity of a stimulus once it is received, to achieve optimum processing for perception and well-being.

Sensory modulation disorder   Malfunctioning of sensory modulation that results in a state of hypo-arousal, hyper-arousal, or inappropriate fluctuation of levels of arousal.

Serotonin   Neurotransmitter which regulates feelings of well-being – implicated in persons with depression or anxiety states.

SIB- Self-Injurious Behaviour   Can range from head-banging, slapping, gouging, hair-plucking, - to life-threatening actions.

SIBIS   Self-Injurious Behaviour Inhibiting System. Notably used when the behaviour has become life-threatening. A helmet which registers a head-bang and delivers a mild shock to the arm.

SLP / SLT   Speech and Language Pathologist / Therapist.

Social Stories   Carol Gray of Jennison County, USA, introduced the method of using written or spoken stories to teach appropriate social behaviours and problem-solving strategies to verbal people with autism.

Son-Rise Also known as the Option Programme. Barry and Sahmaria Kaufmann developed this approach to bring their son Raun from autism. They teach this approach and philosophy at their Institute and abroad.

SLI Specific Language Impairment

SSS see Scotopic Sensitivity Syndrome.

Sulfation The process by which PST attaches sulphur to the phenolic compound.

Super-Nu Thera A comprehensive vitamin-mineral supplement specifically produced to the requirements of children and adults with autism, which is also colour-free, sugar and flavourant-free. Produced by Kirkman Laboratories.

TEACCH Treatment and Education of Autistic and Related Communication-Handicapped Children. A system evolved by Mesibov and Schopler, to structure the learning environment and task, to bring more predictability into the situation and to facilitate the emergence of prompt- independence.

Temporal lobe The part of the brain to the side of the frontal lobes.

Theory of Mind Proposed by Baron-Cohen, emphasising the inability to see situations from another's' point of view, a lack of empathy, as being one of the key features of autism.

Therapeutic Listening A variant of the Tomatis Sound therapy.

Thymus gland Gland behind sternum, which holds a memory of all diseases ever encountered by the body. Malfunctions when persons suffer from myasthenia gravis, when the body "remembers" fictitious diseases and goes about destroying parts of itself in order to eradicate the disease.

TLA Training in Learning Aptitude – like ABA but of different origins, specifically focusing on developing the skills for Communication.

TMG Tri-methyl glycine – the 'big brother' of DMG. Especially useful in cardio-vascular conditions.

Tomatis Sound Therapy Also called the electronic ear. The original auditory technique using electronically modulated music to encourage better listening. This system has strong psychoanalytical overtones, as the system was devised to cure language disorders through maternal bonding by using 'uterine-like' sounds. Used to require 100 hours of listening, several times in succession.

Tourette's syndrome A neurological condition characterised by repetitive, explosive behaviours, or 'tics'. Frequently associated with personality disorders , challenging behaviours and learning disabilities or dyslexia.

Trace Minerals All tissues and internal fluids of our body contain varying quantities of minerals, which are vital to overall mental and physical well-being. Minerals act as catalysts for many biological reactions within the body, including muscle response, the transmission of messages through the nervous system.

Triad of Impairments Dr Lorna Wing's concept of the characteristics of autism:-

Urinary peptide analysis The assessment of the peptide content of urine samples (by Neurozym, Norway; Sunderland, UK; or Great Plains, USA). Gives a quantitative analysis of the severity of the gluten/casein/gliadin intolerance.

Vaccine damage Injury due to adverse reaction to administration of a vaccine. Can range from mild reaction to severe damage, even death.

Verbal-Auditory Agnosia See Auditory Verbal Agnosia.

Vineland Adaptive Behaviour Scales An assessment format to identify social skills requiring intervention.

VMI   Visuo-motor integration.

Visual-motor learning disability   A sub-set of specific learning disabilities / dyslexia, characterised by visual spatial difficulties and poor performance on visual perceptual and fine motor co-ordination tasks

Waldorf – Rudolf Steiner   A philosophy based on the anthroposophical religion. They have schools and resi-dential units for people with learning disabilities. High-functioning people with autism may be admitted, depending on the severity of their challenging behaviours.

Welsh Method   Holding Therapy, or Direct Affective Synchronous Bonding

Yoked prisms   Optic prism lenses put into frames to be worn as part of an exercise programme. Sometimes used in sports, and applied by Melvyn Kaplan to autism and other disorders, e.g. psychiatric conditions, dyslexia.

Young autism project   The 1974 study by Dr Ivar Lovaas into the effectiveness of ABA in autism.

2006

January
S	M	Tu	W	Th	F	S
1	2	3	4	5	6	7
8	9	10	11	12	13	14
15	16	17	18	19	20	21
22	23	24	25	26	27	28
29	30	31				

February
S	M	Tu	W	Th	F	S
			1	2	3	4
5	6	7	8	9	10	11
12	13	14	15	16	17	18
19	20	21	22	23	24	25
26	27	28				

March
S	M	Tu	W	Th	F	S
			1	2	3	4
5	6	7	8	9	10	11
12	13	14	15	16	17	18
19	20	21	22	23	24	25
26	27	28	29	30	31	

April
S	M	Tu	W	Th	F	S
						1
2	3	4	5	6	7	8
9	10	11	12	13	14	15
16	17	18	19	20	21	22
23	24	25	26	27	28	29
30						

May
S	M	Tu	W	Th	F	S
	1	2	3	4	5	6
7	8	9	10	11	12	13
14	15	16	17	18	19	20
21	22	23	24	25	26	27
28	29	30	31			

June
S	M	Tu	W	Th	F	S
				1	2	3
4	5	6	7	8	9	10
11	12	13	14	15	16	17
18	19	20	21	22	23	24
25	26	27	28	29	30	

July
S	M	Tu	W	Th	F	S
						1
2	3	4	5	6	7	8
9	10	11	12	13	14	15
16	17	18	19	20	21	22
23	24	25	26	27	28	29
30	31					

August
S	M	Tu	W	Th	F	S
		1	2	3	4	5
6	7	8	9	10	11	12
13	14	15	16	17	18	19
20	21	22	23	24	25	26
27	28	29	30	31		

September
S	M	Tu	W	Th	F	S
					1	2
3	4	5	6	7	8	9
10	11	12	13	14	15	16
17	18	19	20	21	22	23
24	25	26	27	28	29	30

October
S	M	Tu	W	Th	F	S
1	2	3	4	5	6	7
8	9	10	11	12	13	14
15	16	17	18	19	20	21
22	23	24	25	26	27	28
29	30	31				

November
S	M	Tu	W	Th	F	S
			1	2	3	4
5	6	7	8	9	10	11
12	13	14	15	16	17	18
19	20	21	22	23	24	25
26	27	28	29	30		

December
S	M	Tu	W	Th	F	S
					1	2
3	4	5	6	7	8	9
10	11	12	13	14	15	16
17	18	19	20	21	22	23
24	25	26	27	28	29	30
31						

2006 year planner

January	February	March
April	May	June
July	August	September
October	November	December

Events Record
2006
January
February
March
April
May
June
July
August
September
October
November
December

Use this space to record major events, e.g. breakthroughs, ATEC scores, Neuro-Biological test results, etc..

2007

January
S	M	Tu	W	Th	F	S
	1	2	3	4	5	6
7	8	9	10	11	12	13
14	15	16	17	18	19	20
21	22	23	24	25	26	27
28	29	30	31			

February
S	M	Tu	W	Th	F	S
				1	2	3
4	5	6	7	8	9	10
11	12	13	14	15	16	17
18	19	20	21	22	23	24
25	26	27	28			

March
S	M	Tu	W	Th	F	S
				1	2	3
4	5	6	7	8	9	10
11	12	13	14	15	16	17
18	19	20	21	22	23	24
25	26	27	28	29	30	31

April
S	M	Tu	W	Th	F	S
1	2	3	4	5	6	7
8	9	10	11	12	13	14
15	16	17	18	19	20	21
22	23	24	25	26	27	28
29	30					

May
S	M	Tu	W	Th	F	S
		1	2	3	4	5
6	7	8	9	10	11	12
13	14	15	16	17	18	19
20	21	22	23	24	25	26
27	28	29	30	31		

June
S	M	Tu	W	Th	F	S
					1	2
3	4	5	6	7	8	9
10	11	12	13	14	15	16
17	18	19	20	21	22	23
24	25	26	27	28	29	30

July
S	M	Tu	W	Th	F	S
1	2	3	4	5	6	7
8	9	10	11	12	13	14
15	16	17	18	19	20	21
22	23	24	25	26	27	28
29	30	31				

August
S	M	Tu	W	Th	F	S
			1	2	3	4
5	6	7	8	9	10	11
12	13	14	15	16	17	18
19	20	21	22	23	24	25
26	27	28	29	30	31	

September
S	M	Tu	W	Th	F	S
						1
2	3	4	5	6	7	8
9	10	11	12	13	14	15
16	17	18	19	20	21	22
23	24	25	26	27	28	29
30						

October
S	M	Tu	W	Th	F	S
	1	2	3	4	5	6
7	8	9	10	11	12	13
14	15	16	17	18	19	20
21	22	23	24	25	26	27
28	29	30	31			

November
S	M	Tu	W	Th	F	S
				1	2	3
4	5	6	7	8	9	10
11	12	13	14	15	16	17
18	19	20	21	22	23	24
25	26	27	28	29	30	

December
S	M	Tu	W	Th	F	S
						1
2	3	4	5	6	7	8
9	10	11	12	13	14	15
16	17	18	19	20	21	22
23	24	25	26	27	28	29
30	31					

2007 year planner

January	February	March

April	May	June

July	August	September

October	November	December

Events Record
2007

January	
February	
March	
April	
May	
June	
July	
August	
September	
October	
November	
December	

Use this space to record major events, e.g. breakthroughs, ATEC scores, Neuro-Biological test results, etc..

ABOUT THE AUTHOR

Rosalie Seymour has more than 25 years of experience in this field and has developed a variety of related skills. She is a Bérard Auditory Integration Training practitioner and trainer in the method, and has developed *Training in Learning Aptitude* and *Neuro-Cognitive Mobilisation*. She has written and produced programmes including 'Sounds Right' – a phonics training home programme that was approved by the Cape Education Department.

She writes: " There was a time when I took my information from the people around me, professionals to whom I looked for direction and update. Then in 1993 I attended some conferences that 'blew the lid off' my mind through exposure to the wealth of information available. It was an intensely painful experience to realise that I had been kept in the dark and thereby in a state of blissful *'don't rock the boat'* mediocrity."

Since this experience, she has dedicated her time and effort to operating a resource facility for parents and professionals, running seminars and conferences, holding training courses, and generally making public and available these new developments.

www.ingramcontent.com/pod-product-compliance
Lightning Source LLC
Chambersburg PA
CBHW031230280526
45784CB00004B/1518